THIS BOOK BELONGS TO

____

Date

How are you feeling today?

<table>
<tr><td>

I have eaten...

BREAKFAST	**WHAT TIME?**	Calories

LUNCH	**WHAT TIME?**	Calories

DINNER	**WHAT TIME?**	Calories

SNACKS	**WHAT TIME?**	Calories

TOTAL CALORIES

Weight today?

</td><td>

I have exercised...

DOING?	**TIME**	Calories Burned

**TOTAL CALORIES
BURNED**

I have slept...

HOURS

I have drank...

CUPS OF
WATER

Meds/vitamins taken

FINAL CALORIES
(Calories eaten - calories burned)

Change? +/-

</td></tr>
</table>

Date

How are you feeling today?

I have eaten...

BREAKFAST	**WHAT TIME?**	Calories

LUNCH	**WHAT TIME?**	Calories

DINNER	**WHAT TIME?**	Calories

SNACKS	**WHAT TIME?**	Calories

TOTAL CALORIES

Weight today?

I have exercised...

DOING?	**TIME**	Calories Burned

TOTAL CALORIES BURNED

I have slept...

HOURS

I have drank...

CUPS OF WATER

Meds/vitamins taken

FINAL CALORIES
(Calories eaten - calories burned)

Change? +/-

Date

How are you feeling today?

I have eaten...

BREAKFAST	**WHAT TIME?**	Calories

LUNCH	**WHAT TIME?**	Calories

DINNER	**WHAT TIME?**	Calories

SNACKS	**WHAT TIME?**	Calories

TOTAL CALORIES

Weight today?

I have exercised...

DOING?	**TIME**	Calories Burned

**TOTAL CALORIES
BURNED**

I have slept...

HOURS

I have drank...

CUPS OF
WATER

Meds/vitamins taken

FINAL CALORIES

(Calories eaten - calories burned)

Change? +/-

Date

How are you feeling today?

I have eaten...

| BREAKFAST | **WHAT TIME?** | Calories |

| LUNCH | **WHAT TIME?** | Calories |

| DINNER | **WHAT TIME?** | Calories |

| SNACKS | **WHAT TIME?** | Calories |

TOTAL CALORIES

Weight today?

I have exercised...

| DOING? | **TIME** | Calories Burned |

TOTAL CALORIES BURNED

I have slept...

HOURS

I have drank...

CUPS OF WATER

Meds/vitamins taken

FINAL CALORIES
(Calories eaten - calories burned)

Change? +/-

Date

How are you feeling today?

I have eaten...

BREAKFAST	**WHAT TIME?**	Calories

LUNCH	**WHAT TIME?**	Calories

DINNER	**WHAT TIME?**	Calories

SNACKS	**WHAT TIME?**	Calories

TOTAL CALORIES

Weight today?

I have exercised...

DOING?	**TIME**	Calories Burned

TOTAL CALORIES BURNED

I have slept...

HOURS

I have drank...

CUPS OF WATER

Meds/vitamins taken

FINAL CALORIES

(Calories eaten - calories burned)

Change? +/-

Date

How are you feeling today?

I have eaten...

BREAKFAST   **WHAT TIME?**   Calories

LUNCH   **WHAT TIME?**   Calories

DINNER   **WHAT TIME?**   Calories

SNACKS   **WHAT TIME?**   Calories

TOTAL CALORIES

Weight today?

I have exercised...

DOING?   **TIME**   Calories Burned

TOTAL CALORIES BURNED

I have slept...

HOURS

I have drank...

CUPS OF WATER

Meds/vitamins taken

FINAL CALORIES
(Calories eaten - calories burned)

Change? +/-

Date _______________

How are you feeling today? _______________

I have eaten...

BREAKFAST	**WHAT TIME?**	Calories

LUNCH	**WHAT TIME?**	Calories

DINNER	**WHAT TIME?**	Calories

SNACKS	**WHAT TIME?**	Calories

TOTAL CALORIES _______________

Weight today? _______________

I have exercised...

DOING?	**TIME**	Calories Burned

TOTAL CALORIES BURNED _______________

I have slept...

_______________ HOURS

I have drank...

_______________ CUPS OF WATER

Meds/vitamins taken

FINAL CALORIES _______________
(Calories eaten - calories burned)

Change? +/- _______________

Date _______________________

How are you feeling today? _______________________

I have eaten...

BREAKFAST	**WHAT TIME?**	Calories
LUNCH	**WHAT TIME?**	Calories
DINNER	**WHAT TIME?**	Calories
SNACKS	**WHAT TIME?**	Calories

TOTAL CALORIES _______________________

I have exercised...

DOING?	**TIME**	Calories Burned

TOTAL CALORIES BURNED _______________________

I have slept...

_______________________ HOURS

I have drank...

_______________________ CUPS OF WATER

Meds/vitamins taken

____

____

____

____

FINAL CALORIES _______________________
(Calories eaten - calories burned)

Weight today? _______________________

Change? +/- _______________________

Date

How are you feeling today?

I have eaten...

BREAKFAST	WHAT TIME?	Calories

LUNCH	WHAT TIME?	Calories

DINNER	WHAT TIME?	Calories

SNACKS	WHAT TIME?	Calories

TOTAL CALORIES

Weight today?

I have exercised...

DOING?	TIME	Calories Burned

**TOTAL CALORIES
BURNED**

I have slept...

HOURS

I have drank...

CUPS OF
WATER

Meds/vitamins taken

FINAL CALORIES
(Calories eaten - calories burned)

Change? +/-

Date

How are you feeling today?

<table>
<tr><td>

I have eaten...

BREAKFAST	**WHAT TIME?**	Calories

LUNCH	**WHAT TIME?**	Calories

DINNER	**WHAT TIME?**	Calories

SNACKS	**WHAT TIME?**	Calories

TOTAL CALORIES

</td><td>

I have exercised...

DOING?	**TIME**	Calories Burned

TOTAL CALORIES BURNED

I have slept...

HOURS

I have drank...

CUPS OF WATER

Meds/vitamins taken

FINAL CALORIES
(Calories eaten - calories burned)

</td></tr>
</table>

Weight today?

Change? +/-

Date _______________

How are you feeling today? _______________

I have eaten...

BREAKFAST	**WHAT TIME?**	Calories

LUNCH	**WHAT TIME?**	Calories

DINNER	**WHAT TIME?**	Calories

SNACKS	**WHAT TIME?**	Calories

TOTAL CALORIES _______________

I have exercised...

DOING?	**TIME**	Calories Burned

TOTAL CALORIES BURNED _______________

I have slept...

_______________ HOURS

I have drank...

_______________ CUPS OF WATER

Meds/vitamins taken

____

____

____

FINAL CALORIES _______________
(Calories eaten - calories burned)

Weight today? _______________   **Change? +/-** _______________

Date

How are you feeling today?

I have eaten...			I have exercised...		
BREAKFAST	WHAT TIME?	Calories	DOING?	TIME	Calories Burned
LUNCH	WHAT TIME?	Calories			
DINNER	WHAT TIME?	Calories	**TOTAL CALORIES BURNED**		

I have slept...

HOURS

I have drank...

CUPS OF WATER

Meds/vitamins taken

SNACKS	WHAT TIME?	Calories

TOTAL CALORIES

FINAL CALORIES

(Calories eaten - calories burned)

Weight today?

Change? +/-

Date _______________________

How are you feeling today? _______________________

I have eaten...

BREAKFAST	**WHAT TIME?**	Calories

I have exercised...

DOING?	**TIME**	Calories Burned

LUNCH	**WHAT TIME?**	Calories

TOTAL CALORIES BURNED _______________________

I have slept...

_______________________ HOURS

DINNER	**WHAT TIME?**	Calories

I have drank...

_______________________ CUPS OF WATER

Meds/vitamins taken

SNACKS	**WHAT TIME?**	Calories

TOTAL CALORIES _______________________

FINAL CALORIES _______________________
(Calories eaten - calories burned)

Weight today? _______________________

Change? +/- _______________________

Date

How are you feeling today?

I have eaten...

BREAKFAST	WHAT TIME?	Calories

LUNCH	WHAT TIME?	Calories

DINNER	WHAT TIME?	Calories

SNACKS	WHAT TIME?	Calories

TOTAL CALORIES

I have exercised...

DOING?	TIME	Calories Burned

TOTAL CALORIES BURNED

I have slept...

HOURS

I have drank...

CUPS OF WATER

Meds/vitamins taken

FINAL CALORIES

(Calories eaten - calories burned)

Weight today?

Change? +/-

Date _______________________

How are you feeling today? _______________________

I have eaten...

BREAKFAST	**WHAT TIME?**	Calories

LUNCH	**WHAT TIME?**	Calories

DINNER	**WHAT TIME?**	Calories

SNACKS	**WHAT TIME?**	Calories

TOTAL CALORIES _______________________

Weight today? _______________________

I have exercised...

DOING?	**TIME**	Calories Burned

TOTAL CALORIES BURNED _______________________

I have slept...

_______________________ HOURS

I have drank...

_______________________ CUPS OF WATER

Meds/vitamins taken

____

____

____

____

FINAL CALORIES _______________________
(Calories eaten - calories burned)

Change? +/- _______________________

Date

How are you feeling today?

I have eaten...

BREAKFAST	WHAT TIME?	Calories

LUNCH	WHAT TIME?	Calories

DINNER	WHAT TIME?	Calories

SNACKS	WHAT TIME?	Calories

TOTAL CALORIES

Weight today?

I have exercised...

DOING?	TIME	Calories Burned

TOTAL CALORIES BURNED

I have slept...

HOURS

I have drank...

CUPS OF WATER

Meds/vitamins taken

FINAL CALORIES
(Calories eaten - calories burned)

Change? +/-

Date ____________________

How are you feeling today? ____________________

I have eaten...

BREAKFAST	**WHAT TIME?**	Calories

LUNCH	**WHAT TIME?**	Calories

DINNER	**WHAT TIME?**	Calories

SNACKS	**WHAT TIME?**	Calories

TOTAL CALORIES ______________

Weight today? ______________

I have exercised...

DOING?	**TIME**	Calories Burned

TOTAL CALORIES BURNED ______________

I have slept...

______________ HOURS

I have drank...

______________ CUPS OF WATER

Meds/vitamins taken

FINAL CALORIES ______________
(Calories eaten - calories burned)

Change? +/- ______________

Date ___________________

How are you feeling today? ___________________

I have eaten...
I have exercised...

BREAKFAST	**WHAT TIME?**	Calories

DOING?	**TIME**	Calories Burned

LUNCH	**WHAT TIME?**	Calories

TOTAL CALORIES BURNED ___________________

I have slept...
HOURS ___________________

DINNER	**WHAT TIME?**	Calories

I have drank...
CUPS OF WATER ___________________

Meds/vitamins taken

SNACKS	**WHAT TIME?**	Calories

TOTAL CALORIES ___________________

FINAL CALORIES ___________________
(Calories eaten - calories burned)

Weight today? ___________________

Change? +/- ___________________

Date

How are you feeling today?

I have eaten...

BREAKFAST	**WHAT TIME?**	Calories

LUNCH	**WHAT TIME?**	Calories

DINNER	**WHAT TIME?**	Calories

SNACKS	**WHAT TIME?**	Calories

TOTAL CALORIES

Weight today?

I have exercised...

DOING?	**TIME**	Calories Burned

TOTAL CALORIES BURNED

I have slept...

HOURS

I have drank...

CUPS OF WATER

Meds/vitamins taken

FINAL CALORIES
(Calories eaten - calories burned)

Change? +/-

Date

How are you feeling today?

I have eaten...

BREAKFAST	**WHAT TIME?**	Calories

LUNCH	**WHAT TIME?**	Calories

DINNER	**WHAT TIME?**	Calories

SNACKS	**WHAT TIME?**	Calories

TOTAL CALORIES

Weight today?

I have exercised...

DOING?	**TIME**	Calories Burned

TOTAL CALORIES BURNED

I have slept...

HOURS

I have drank...

CUPS OF WATER

Meds/vitamins taken

FINAL CALORIES
(Calories eaten - calories burned)

Change? +/-

Date _______________

How are you feeling today? _______________

I have eaten...

BREAKFAST	**WHAT TIME?**	Calories

LUNCH	**WHAT TIME?**	Calories

DINNER	**WHAT TIME?**	Calories

SNACKS	**WHAT TIME?**	Calories

TOTAL CALORIES _______________

Weight today? _______________

I have exercised...

DOING?	**TIME**	Calories Burned

TOTAL CALORIES BURNED _______________

I have slept...

_______________ HOURS

I have drank...

_______________ CUPS OF WATER

Meds/vitamins taken

FINAL CALORIES _______________
(Calories eaten - calories burned)

Change? +/- _______________

Date

How are you feeling today?

I have eaten...

| BREAKFAST | **WHAT TIME?** | Calories |

| LUNCH | **WHAT TIME?** | Calories |

| DINNER | **WHAT TIME?** | Calories |

| SNACKS | **WHAT TIME?** | Calories |

TOTAL CALORIES

Weight today?

I have exercised...

| DOING? | **TIME** | Calories Burned |

TOTAL CALORIES BURNED

I have slept...

HOURS

I have drank...

CUPS OF WATER

Meds/vitamins taken

FINAL CALORIES

(Calories eaten - calories burned)

Change? +/-

Date ______________________

How are you feeling today? ______________________

I have eaten...

BREAKFAST	**WHAT TIME?**	Calories

LUNCH	**WHAT TIME?**	Calories

DINNER	**WHAT TIME?**	Calories

SNACKS	**WHAT TIME?**	Calories

TOTAL CALORIES ______________________

Weight today? ______________________

I have exercised...

DOING?	**TIME**	Calories Burned

TOTAL CALORIES BURNED ______________________

I have slept...

HOURS ______________________

I have drank...

CUPS OF WATER ______________________

Meds/vitamins taken

FINAL CALORIES ______________________
(Calories eaten - calories burned)

Change? +/- ______________________

Date

How are you feeling today?

I have eaten...

BREAKFAST	**WHAT TIME?**	Calories

LUNCH	**WHAT TIME?**	Calories

DINNER	**WHAT TIME?**	Calories

SNACKS	**WHAT TIME?**	Calories

TOTAL CALORIES

Weight today?

I have exercised...

DOING?	**TIME**	Calories Burned

TOTAL CALORIES BURNED

I have slept...

HOURS

I have drank...

CUPS OF WATER

Meds/vitamins taken

FINAL CALORIES

(Calories eaten - calories burned)

Change? +/-

Date

How are you feeling today?

I have eaten...

BREAKFAST	**WHAT TIME?**	Calories

LUNCH	**WHAT TIME?**	Calories

DINNER	**WHAT TIME?**	Calories

SNACKS	**WHAT TIME?**	Calories

TOTAL CALORIES

Weight today?

I have exercised...

DOING?	**TIME**	Calories Burned

TOTAL CALORIES BURNED

I have slept...

HOURS

I have drank...

CUPS OF WATER

Meds/vitamins taken

FINAL CALORIES

(Calories eaten - calories burned)

Change? +/-

Date _______________________

How are you feeling today? _______________________

<table>
<tr><td>

I have eaten...

</td><td>

I have exercised...

</td></tr>
</table>

BREAKFAST	**WHAT TIME?**	Calories

DOING?	**TIME**	Calories Burned

LUNCH	**WHAT TIME?**	Calories

TOTAL CALORIES BURNED _______________________

I have slept...

HOURS

DINNER	**WHAT TIME?**	Calories

I have drank...

CUPS OF WATER

Meds/vitamins taken

SNACKS	**WHAT TIME?**	Calories

TOTAL CALORIES _______________________

FINAL CALORIES _______________________
(Calories eaten - calories burned)

Weight today? _______________________

Change? +/- _______________________

Date _______________

How are you feeling today? _______________

I have eaten...

BREAKFAST	**WHAT TIME?**	Calories

LUNCH	**WHAT TIME?**	Calories

DINNER	**WHAT TIME?**	Calories

SNACKS	**WHAT TIME?**	Calories

TOTAL CALORIES

Weight today? _______________

I have exercised...

DOING?	**TIME**	Calories Burned

TOTAL CALORIES BURNED _______________

I have slept...

_______________ HOURS

I have drank...

_______________ CUPS OF WATER

Meds/vitamins taken

FINAL CALORIES _______________
(Calories eaten - calories burned)

Change? +/- _______________

Date

How are you feeling today?

I have eaten...

BREAKFAST	**WHAT TIME?**	Calories

LUNCH	**WHAT TIME?**	Calories

DINNER	**WHAT TIME?**	Calories

SNACKS	**WHAT TIME?**	Calories

TOTAL CALORIES

Weight today?

I have exercised...

DOING?	**TIME**	Calories Burned

TOTAL CALORIES BURNED

I have slept...

HOURS

I have drank...

CUPS OF WATER

Meds/vitamins taken

FINAL CALORIES

(Calories eaten - calories burned)

Change? +/-

Date _______________

How are you feeling today? _______________

I have eaten...

BREAKFAST	WHAT TIME?	Calories

LUNCH	WHAT TIME?	Calories

DINNER	WHAT TIME?	Calories

SNACKS	WHAT TIME?	Calories

TOTAL CALORIES _______________

Weight today? _______________

I have exercised...

DOING?	TIME	Calories Burned

TOTAL CALORIES BURNED _______________

I have slept...

_______________ HOURS

I have drank...

_______________ CUPS OF WATER

Meds/vitamins taken

____

FINAL CALORIES _______________
(Calories eaten - calories burned)

Change? +/- _______________

Date _______________

How are you feeling today? _______________

I have eaten...

BREAKFAST	**WHAT TIME?**	Calories

LUNCH	**WHAT TIME?**	Calories

DINNER	**WHAT TIME?**	Calories

SNACKS	**WHAT TIME?**	Calories

TOTAL CALORIES _______________

Weight today? _______________

I have exercised...

DOING?	**TIME**	Calories Burned

TOTAL CALORIES BURNED _______________

I have slept...

_______________ HOURS

I have drank...

_______________ CUPS OF WATER

Meds/vitamins taken

FINAL CALORIES _______________
(Calories eaten - calories burned)

Change? +/- _______________

Date _______________

How are you feeling today? _______________

I have eaten...   # I have exercised...

| BREAKFAST | **WHAT TIME?** | Calories |

| DOING? | **TIME** | Calories Burned |

| LUNCH | **WHAT TIME?** | Calories |

**TOTAL CALORIES
BURNED** _______________

I have slept...

HOURS

| DINNER | **WHAT TIME?** | Calories |

I have drank...

CUPS OF
WATER

Meds/vitamins taken

| SNACKS | **WHAT TIME?** | Calories |

TOTAL CALORIES _______________

FINAL CALORIES _______________
(Calories eaten - calories burned)

Weight today? _______________   # Change? +/- _______________

Date ______________________

How are you feeling today? ______________________

<table>
<tr><td colspan="3"># I have eaten...</td><td colspan="3"># I have exercised...</td></tr>
<tr><td>BREAKFAST</td><td>WHAT TIME?</td><td>Calories</td><td>DOING?</td><td>TIME</td><td>Calories Burned</td></tr>
</table>

I have eaten...

BREAKFAST	WHAT TIME?	Calories

LUNCH	WHAT TIME?	Calories

DINNER	WHAT TIME?	Calories

SNACKS	WHAT TIME?	Calories

TOTAL CALORIES ______________________

Weight today? ______________________

I have exercised...

DOING?	TIME	Calories Burned

TOTAL CALORIES BURNED ______________________

I have slept...

______________________ HOURS

I have drank...

______________________ CUPS OF WATER

Meds/vitamins taken

____

____

____

FINAL CALORIES ______________________
(Calories eaten - calories burned)

Change? +/- ______________________

Date _______________

How are you feeling today? _______________

I have eaten...

BREAKFAST	**WHAT TIME?**	Calories

LUNCH	**WHAT TIME?**	Calories

DINNER	**WHAT TIME?**	Calories

SNACKS	**WHAT TIME?**	Calories

TOTAL CALORIES _______________

Weight today? _______________

I have exercised...

DOING?	**TIME**	Calories Burned

TOTAL CALORIES BURNED _______________

I have slept...

_______________ HOURS

I have drank...

_______________ CUPS OF WATER

Meds/vitamins taken

FINAL CALORIES _______________
(Calories eaten - calories burned)

Change? +/- _______________

Date

How are you feeling today?

I have eaten...

BREAKFAST	**WHAT TIME?**	Calories

LUNCH	**WHAT TIME?**	Calories

DINNER	**WHAT TIME?**	Calories

SNACKS	**WHAT TIME?**	Calories

TOTAL CALORIES

Weight today?

I have exercised...

DOING?	**TIME**	Calories Burned

TOTAL CALORIES BURNED

I have slept...

HOURS

I have drank...

CUPS OF WATER

Meds/vitamins taken

FINAL CALORIES
(Calories eaten - calories burned)

Change? +/-

Date _______________________

How are you feeling today? _______________________

I have eaten...

BREAKFAST	**WHAT TIME?**	Calories

LUNCH	**WHAT TIME?**	Calories

DINNER	**WHAT TIME?**	Calories

SNACKS	**WHAT TIME?**	Calories

TOTAL CALORIES _______________________

Weight today? _______________________

I have exercised...

DOING?	**TIME**	Calories Burned

TOTAL CALORIES BURNED _______________________

I have slept...

_______________________ HOURS

I have drank...

_______________________ CUPS OF WATER

Meds/vitamins taken

FINAL CALORIES _______________________
(Calories eaten - calories burned)

Change? +/- _______________________

Date

How are you feeling today?

I have eaten...

| BREAKFAST | **WHAT TIME?** | Calories |

| LUNCH | **WHAT TIME?** | Calories |

| DINNER | **WHAT TIME?** | Calories |

| SNACKS | **WHAT TIME?** | Calories |

TOTAL CALORIES

Weight today?

I have exercised...

| DOING? | **TIME** | Calories Burned |

**TOTAL CALORIES
BURNED**

I have slept...

HOURS

I have drank...

CUPS OF
WATER

Meds/vitamins taken

FINAL CALORIES
(Calories eaten - calories burned)

Change? +/-

Date ______________________

How are you feeling today? ______________________

I have eaten...   ## I have exercised...

BREAKFAST	**WHAT TIME?**	Calories

DOING?	**TIME**	Calories Burned

LUNCH	**WHAT TIME?**	Calories

TOTAL CALORIES BURNED ______________________

I have slept...

HOURS ______________________

DINNER	**WHAT TIME?**	Calories

I have drank...

CUPS OF WATER

Meds/vitamins taken

SNACKS	**WHAT TIME?**	Calories

TOTAL CALORIES ______________________

FINAL CALORIES ______________________
(Calories eaten - calories burned)

Weight today? ______________________   ## Change? +/- ______________________

Date

How are you feeling today?

I have eaten...

BREAKFAST	**WHAT TIME?**	Calories

LUNCH	**WHAT TIME?**	Calories

DINNER	**WHAT TIME?**	Calories

SNACKS	**WHAT TIME?**	Calories

TOTAL CALORIES

Weight today?

I have exercised...

DOING?	**TIME**	Calories Burned

**TOTAL CALORIES
BURNED**

I have slept...

HOURS

I have drank...

CUPS OF
WATER

Meds/vitamins taken

FINAL CALORIES

(Calories eaten - calories burned)

Change? +/-

Date

How are you feeling today?

I have eaten...

BREAKFAST	**WHAT TIME?**	Calories

LUNCH	**WHAT TIME?**	Calories

DINNER	**WHAT TIME?**	Calories

SNACKS	**WHAT TIME?**	Calories

TOTAL CALORIES

Weight today?

I have exercised...

DOING?	**TIME**	Calories Burned

TOTAL CALORIES BURNED

I have slept...

HOURS

I have drank...

CUPS OF WATER

Meds/vitamins taken

FINAL CALORIES

(Calories eaten - calories burned)

Change? +/-

Date

How are you feeling today?

I have eaten...

BREAKFAST	**WHAT TIME?**	Calories

LUNCH	**WHAT TIME?**	Calories

DINNER	**WHAT TIME?**	Calories

SNACKS	**WHAT TIME?**	Calories

TOTAL CALORIES

Weight today?

I have exercised...

DOING?	**TIME**	Calories Burned

TOTAL CALORIES BURNED

I have slept...

HOURS

I have drank...

CUPS OF WATER

Meds/vitamins taken

FINAL CALORIES

(Calories eaten - calories burned)

Change? +/-

Date

How are you feeling today?

I have eaten...

| BREAKFAST | **WHAT TIME?** | Calories |

| LUNCH | **WHAT TIME?** | Calories |

| DINNER | **WHAT TIME?** | Calories |

| SNACKS | **WHAT TIME?** | Calories |

TOTAL CALORIES

Weight today?

I have exercised...

| DOING? | **TIME** | Calories Burned |

TOTAL CALORIES BURNED

I have slept...

HOURS

I have drank...

CUPS OF WATER

Meds/vitamins taken

FINAL CALORIES

(Calories eaten - calories burned)

Change? +/-

Date

How are you feeling today?

I have eaten...

BREAKFAST	**WHAT TIME?**	Calories

LUNCH	**WHAT TIME?**	Calories

DINNER	**WHAT TIME?**	Calories

SNACKS	**WHAT TIME?**	Calories

TOTAL CALORIES

Weight today?

I have exercised...

DOING?	**TIME**	Calories Burned

TOTAL CALORIES BURNED

I have slept...

HOURS

I have drank...

CUPS OF WATER

Meds/vitamins taken

FINAL CALORIES
(Calories eaten - calories burned)

Change? +/-

Date ______________________

How are you feeling today? ______________________

I have eaten...

BREAKFAST	**WHAT TIME?**	Calories

LUNCH	**WHAT TIME?**	Calories

DINNER	**WHAT TIME?**	Calories

SNACKS	**WHAT TIME?**	Calories

TOTAL CALORIES ______________________

Weight today? ______________________

I have exercised...

DOING?	**TIME**	Calories Burned

TOTAL CALORIES BURNED ______________________

I have slept...

______________________ HOURS

I have drank...

CUPS OF WATER

Meds/vitamins taken

____

____

____

____

FINAL CALORIES ______________________
(Calories eaten - calories burned)

Change? +/- ______________________

Date

How are you feeling today?

I have eaten...

BREAKFAST	WHAT TIME?	Calories

LUNCH	WHAT TIME?	Calories

DINNER	WHAT TIME?	Calories

SNACKS	WHAT TIME?	Calories

TOTAL CALORIES

Weight today?

I have exercised...

DOING?	TIME	Calories Burned

TOTAL CALORIES BURNED

I have slept...

HOURS

I have drank...

CUPS OF WATER

Meds/vitamins taken

FINAL CALORIES

(Calories eaten - calories burned)

Change? +/-

Date _______________

How are you feeling today? _______________

I have eaten...

BREAKFAST	**WHAT TIME?**	Calories

LUNCH	**WHAT TIME?**	Calories

DINNER	**WHAT TIME?**	Calories

SNACKS	**WHAT TIME?**	Calories

TOTAL CALORIES _______________

Weight today? _______________

I have exercised...

DOING?	**TIME**	Calories Burned

TOTAL CALORIES BURNED _______________

I have slept...

_______________ HOURS

I have drank...

_______________ CUPS OF WATER

Meds/vitamins taken

____

____

____

FINAL CALORIES _______________
(Calories eaten - calories burned)

Change? +/- _______________

Date

How are you feeling today?

I have eaten...

BREAKFAST	**WHAT TIME?**	Calories

LUNCH	**WHAT TIME?**	Calories

DINNER	**WHAT TIME?**	Calories

SNACKS	**WHAT TIME?**	Calories

TOTAL CALORIES

Weight today?

I have exercised...

DOING?	**TIME**	Calories Burned

TOTAL CALORIES BURNED

I have slept...

HOURS

I have drank...

CUPS OF WATER

Meds/vitamins taken

FINAL CALORIES

(Calories eaten - calories burned)

Change? +/-

Date _______________

How are you feeling today? _______________

I have eaten...

BREAKFAST	**WHAT TIME?**	Calories

I have exercised...

DOING?	**TIME**	Calories Burned

LUNCH	**WHAT TIME?**	Calories

TOTAL CALORIES BURNED _______________

I have slept...

_______________ HOURS

DINNER	**WHAT TIME?**	Calories

I have drank...

_______________ CUPS OF WATER

Meds/vitamins taken

SNACKS	**WHAT TIME?**	Calories

TOTAL CALORIES _______________

FINAL CALORIES _______________
(Calories eaten - calories burned)

Weight today? _______________

Change? +/- _______________

Date _______________________

How are you feeling today? _______________________

I have eaten...

BREAKFAST	**WHAT TIME?**	Calories

LUNCH	**WHAT TIME?**	Calories

DINNER	**WHAT TIME?**	Calories

SNACKS	**WHAT TIME?**	Calories

TOTAL CALORIES _______________________

Weight today? _______________________

I have exercised...

DOING?	**TIME**	Calories Burned

TOTAL CALORIES BURNED _______________________

I have slept...

_______________________ HOURS

I have drank...

_______________________ CUPS OF WATER

Meds/vitamins taken

____

FINAL CALORIES _______________________
(Calories eaten - calories burned)

Change? +/- _______________________

Date

How are you feeling today?

I have eaten...

BREAKFAST	WHAT TIME?	Calories

LUNCH	WHAT TIME?	Calories

DINNER	WHAT TIME?	Calories

SNACKS	WHAT TIME?	Calories

TOTAL CALORIES

Weight today?

I have exercised...

DOING?	TIME	Calories Burned

TOTAL CALORIES BURNED

I have slept...

HOURS

I have drank...

CUPS OF WATER

Meds/vitamins taken

FINAL CALORIES

(Calories eaten - calories burned)

Change? +/-

Date

How are you feeling today?

I have eaten...

BREAKFAST	**WHAT TIME?**	Calories

LUNCH	**WHAT TIME?**	Calories

DINNER	**WHAT TIME?**	Calories

SNACKS	**WHAT TIME?**	Calories

TOTAL CALORIES

Weight today?

I have exercised...

DOING?	**TIME**	Calories Burned

TOTAL CALORIES BURNED

I have slept...

HOURS

I have drank...

CUPS OF WATER

Meds/vitamins taken

FINAL CALORIES
(Calories eaten - calories burned)

Change? +/-

Date _______________

How are you feeling today? _______________

<table>
<tr><td>

I have eaten...

BREAKFAST	**WHAT TIME?**	Calories

LUNCH	**WHAT TIME?**	Calories

DINNER	**WHAT TIME?**	Calories

SNACKS	**WHAT TIME?**	Calories

TOTAL CALORIES _______________

Weight today? _______________

</td><td>

I have exercised...

DOING?	**TIME**	Calories Burned

TOTAL CALORIES BURNED _______________

I have slept...

_______________ HOURS

I have drank...

_______________ CUPS OF WATER

Meds/vitamins taken

____

____

____

____

FINAL CALORIES _______________
(Calories eaten - calories burned)

Change? +/- _______________

</td></tr>
</table>

Date

How are you feeling today?

I have eaten...			I have exercised...		
BREAKFAST	**WHAT TIME?**	Calories	DOING?	**TIME**	Calories Burned

TOTAL CALORIES BURNED

LUNCH	**WHAT TIME?**	Calories

I have slept...

HOURS

DINNER	**WHAT TIME?**	Calories

I have drank...

CUPS OF WATER

Meds/vitamins taken

SNACKS	**WHAT TIME?**	Calories

TOTAL CALORIES

FINAL CALORIES

(Calories eaten - calories burned)

Weight today?

Change? +/-

Date

How are you feeling today?

I have eaten...

BREAKFAST	**WHAT TIME?**	Calories

LUNCH	**WHAT TIME?**	Calories

DINNER	**WHAT TIME?**	Calories

SNACKS	**WHAT TIME?**	Calories

TOTAL CALORIES

Weight today?

I have exercised...

DOING?	**TIME**	Calories Burned

**TOTAL CALORIES
BURNED**

I have slept...

HOURS

I have drank...

CUPS OF
WATER

Meds/vitamins taken

FINAL CALORIES

(Calories eaten - calories burned)

Change? +/-

Date

How are you feeling today?

<table>
<tr><td colspan="3">

I have eaten...
</td><td colspan="3">

I have exercised...
</td></tr>
<tr><td>BREAKFAST</td><td>WHAT TIME?</td><td>Calories</td><td>DOING?</td><td>TIME</td><td>Calories Burned</td></tr>
</table>

LUNCH   **WHAT TIME?**   Calories

TOTAL CALORIES BURNED

I have slept...

HOURS

DINNER   **WHAT TIME?**   Calories

I have drank...

CUPS OF WATER

Meds/vitamins taken

SNACKS   **WHAT TIME?**   Calories

TOTAL CALORIES

FINAL CALORIES

(Calories eaten - calories burned)

Weight today?

Change? +/-

Date _______________

How are you feeling today? _______________

I have eaten...

BREAKFAST	WHAT TIME?	Calories

LUNCH	WHAT TIME?	Calories

DINNER	WHAT TIME?	Calories

SNACKS	WHAT TIME?	Calories

TOTAL CALORIES _______________

Weight today? _______________

I have exercised...

DOING?	TIME	Calories Burned

TOTAL CALORIES BURNED _______________

I have slept...

_______________ HOURS

I have drank...

CUPS OF WATER

Meds/vitamins taken

____
____
____
____

FINAL CALORIES _______________
(Calories eaten - calories burned)

Change? +/- _______________

Date

How are you feeling today?

I have eaten...

BREAKFAST	**WHAT TIME?**	Calories

LUNCH	**WHAT TIME?**	Calories

DINNER	**WHAT TIME?**	Calories

SNACKS	**WHAT TIME?**	Calories

TOTAL CALORIES

Weight today?

I have exercised...

DOING?	**TIME**	Calories Burned

TOTAL CALORIES BURNED

I have slept...

HOURS

I have drank...

CUPS OF WATER

Meds/vitamins taken

FINAL CALORIES
(Calories eaten - calories burned)

Change? +/-

Date

How are you feeling today?

I have eaten...

BREAKFAST	**WHAT TIME?**	Calories

LUNCH	**WHAT TIME?**	Calories

DINNER	**WHAT TIME?**	Calories

SNACKS	**WHAT TIME?**	Calories

TOTAL CALORIES

Weight today?

I have exercised...

DOING?	**TIME**	Calories Burned

TOTAL CALORIES BURNED

I have slept...

HOURS

I have drank...

CUPS OF WATER

Meds/vitamins taken

FINAL CALORIES

(Calories eaten - calories burned)

Change? +/-

Date

How are you feeling today?

I have eaten...

BREAKFAST	WHAT TIME?	Calories

LUNCH	WHAT TIME?	Calories

DINNER	WHAT TIME?	Calories

SNACKS	WHAT TIME?	Calories

TOTAL CALORIES

Weight today?

I have exercised...

DOING?	TIME	Calories Burned

TOTAL CALORIES BURNED

I have slept...

HOURS

I have drank...

CUPS OF WATER

Meds/vitamins taken

FINAL CALORIES

(Calories eaten - calories burned)

Change? +/-

Date ______________________

How are you feeling today? ______________________

I have eaten...   ## I have exercised...

BREAKFAST	**WHAT TIME?**	Calories

DOING?   **TIME**   Calories Burned

LUNCH	**WHAT TIME?**	Calories

TOTAL CALORIES BURNED ______________________

I have slept...

HOURS

DINNER	**WHAT TIME?**	Calories

I have drank...

CUPS OF WATER

Meds/vitamins taken

SNACKS	**WHAT TIME?**	Calories

TOTAL CALORIES   **FINAL CALORIES**
(Calories eaten - calories burned)

Weight today? ______________   ## Change? +/- ______________

Date

How are you feeling today?

I have eaten...

BREAKFAST	**WHAT TIME?**	Calories

LUNCH	**WHAT TIME?**	Calories

DINNER	**WHAT TIME?**	Calories

SNACKS	**WHAT TIME?**	Calories

TOTAL CALORIES

Weight today?

I have exercised...

DOING?	**TIME**	Calories Burned

TOTAL CALORIES BURNED

I have slept...

HOURS

I have drank...

CUPS OF WATER

Meds/vitamins taken

FINAL CALORIES
(Calories eaten - calories burned)

Change? +/-

Date

How are you feeling today?

I have eaten...

BREAKFAST	**WHAT TIME?**	Calories

LUNCH	**WHAT TIME?**	Calories

DINNER	**WHAT TIME?**	Calories

SNACKS	**WHAT TIME?**	Calories

TOTAL CALORIES

Weight today?

I have exercised...

DOING?	**TIME**	Calories Burned

TOTAL CALORIES BURNED

I have slept...

HOURS

I have drank...

CUPS OF WATER

Meds/vitamins taken

FINAL CALORIES
(Calories eaten - calories burned)

Change? +/-

Date

How are you feeling today?

I have eaten...

| BREAKFAST | **WHAT TIME?** | Calories |

| LUNCH | **WHAT TIME?** | Calories |

| DINNER | **WHAT TIME?** | Calories |

| SNACKS | **WHAT TIME?** | Calories |

TOTAL CALORIES

Weight today?

I have exercised...

| DOING? | **TIME** | Calories Burned |

TOTAL CALORIES BURNED

I have slept...

HOURS

I have drank...

CUPS OF WATER

Meds/vitamins taken

FINAL CALORIES
(Calories eaten - calories burned)

Change? +/-

Date

How are you feeling today?

I have eaten...

| BREAKFAST | **WHAT TIME?** | Calories |

| LUNCH | **WHAT TIME?** | Calories |

| DINNER | **WHAT TIME?** | Calories |

| SNACKS | **WHAT TIME?** | Calories |

TOTAL CALORIES

Weight today?

I have exercised...

| DOING? | **TIME** | Calories Burned |

**TOTAL CALORIES
BURNED**

I have slept...

HOURS

I have drank...

CUPS OF
WATER

Meds/vitamins taken

FINAL CALORIES
(Calories eaten - calories burned)

Change? +/-

Date ______________________

How are you feeling today? ______________________

I have eaten...

BREAKFAST	**WHAT TIME?**	Calories

LUNCH	**WHAT TIME?**	Calories

DINNER	**WHAT TIME?**	Calories

SNACKS	**WHAT TIME?**	Calories

TOTAL CALORIES ______________________

Weight today? ______________________

I have exercised...

DOING?	**TIME**	Calories Burned

TOTAL CALORIES BURNED ______________________

I have slept...

______________________ HOURS

I have drank...

______________________ CUPS OF WATER

Meds/vitamins taken

____

____

____

____

FINAL CALORIES ______________________
(Calories eaten - calories burned)

Change? +/- ______________________

Date

How are you feeling today?

I have eaten...

BREAKFAST	**WHAT TIME?**	Calories

LUNCH	**WHAT TIME?**	Calories

DINNER	**WHAT TIME?**	Calories

SNACKS	**WHAT TIME?**	Calories

TOTAL CALORIES

Weight today?

I have exercised...

DOING?	**TIME**	Calories Burned

**TOTAL CALORIES
BURNED**

I have slept...

HOURS

I have drank...

CUPS OF
WATER

Meds/vitamins taken

FINAL CALORIES

(Calories eaten - calories burned)

Change? +/-

Date _______________________

How are you feeling today? _______________________

<table>
<tr><td colspan="3">

I have eaten...

</td><td colspan="3">

I have exercised...

</td></tr>
<tr><td>BREAKFAST</td><td>**WHAT TIME?**</td><td>Calories</td><td>DOING?</td><td>**TIME**</td><td>Calories Burned</td></tr>
</table>

LUNCH　**WHAT TIME?**　Calories

TOTAL CALORIES BURNED _______________________

I have slept...

HOURS _______________________

DINNER　**WHAT TIME?**　Calories

I have drank...

CUPS OF WATER _______________________

Meds/vitamins taken

SNACKS　**WHAT TIME?**　Calories

TOTAL CALORIES _______________________

FINAL CALORIES _______________________
(Calories eaten - calories burned)

Weight today? _______________________

Change? +/- _______________________

Date

How are you feeling today?

I have eaten...

BREAKFAST	WHAT TIME?	Calories

LUNCH	WHAT TIME?	Calories

DINNER	WHAT TIME?	Calories

SNACKS	WHAT TIME?	Calories

TOTAL CALORIES

Weight today?

I have exercised...

DOING?	TIME	Calories Burned

TOTAL CALORIES BURNED

I have slept...

HOURS

I have drank...

CUPS OF WATER

Meds/vitamins taken

FINAL CALORIES
(Calories eaten - calories burned)

Change? +/-

Date

How are you feeling today?

I have eaten...

BREAKFAST	**WHAT TIME?**	Calories

LUNCH	**WHAT TIME?**	Calories

DINNER	**WHAT TIME?**	Calories

SNACKS	**WHAT TIME?**	Calories

TOTAL CALORIES

Weight today?

I have exercised...

DOING?	**TIME**	Calories Burned

TOTAL CALORIES BURNED

I have slept...

HOURS

I have drank...

CUPS OF WATER

Meds/vitamins taken

FINAL CALORIES
(Calories eaten - calories burned)

Change? +/-

Date _______________________

How are you feeling today? _______________________

I have eaten...

BREAKFAST	**WHAT TIME?**	Calories

LUNCH	**WHAT TIME?**	Calories

DINNER	**WHAT TIME?**	Calories

SNACKS	**WHAT TIME?**	Calories

TOTAL CALORIES _______________________

Weight today? _______________________

I have exercised...

DOING?	**TIME**	Calories Burned

TOTAL CALORIES BURNED _______________________

I have slept...

_______________________ HOURS

I have drank...

CUPS OF WATER

Meds/vitamins taken

____
____
____

FINAL CALORIES _______________________
(Calories eaten - calories burned)

Change? +/- _______________________

Date

How are you feeling today?

I have eaten...

BREAKFAST	**WHAT TIME?**	Calories

LUNCH	**WHAT TIME?**	Calories

DINNER	**WHAT TIME?**	Calories

SNACKS	**WHAT TIME?**	Calories

TOTAL CALORIES

Weight today?

I have exercised...

DOING?	**TIME**	Calories Burned

**TOTAL CALORIES
BURNED**

I have slept...

HOURS

I have drank...

CUPS OF
WATER

Meds/vitamins taken

FINAL CALORIES

(Calories eaten - calories burned)

Change? +/-

Date _______________________

How are you feeling today? _______________________

I have eaten...

BREAKFAST	**WHAT TIME?**	Calories

LUNCH	**WHAT TIME?**	Calories

DINNER	**WHAT TIME?**	Calories

SNACKS	**WHAT TIME?**	Calories

TOTAL CALORIES _______________________

I have exercised...

DOING?	**TIME**	Calories Burned

TOTAL CALORIES BURNED _______________________

I have slept...

_______________________ HOURS

I have drank...

_______________________ CUPS OF WATER

Meds/vitamins taken

____

____

____

FINAL CALORIES _______________________
(Calories eaten - calories burned)

Weight today? _______________________

Change? +/- _______________________

Date

How are you feeling today?

I have eaten...

BREAKFAST	**WHAT TIME?**	Calories

LUNCH	**WHAT TIME?**	Calories

DINNER	**WHAT TIME?**	Calories

SNACKS	**WHAT TIME?**	Calories

TOTAL CALORIES

Weight today?

I have exercised...

DOING?	**TIME**	Calories Burned

**TOTAL CALORIES
BURNED**

I have slept...

HOURS

I have drank...

CUPS OF
WATER

Meds/vitamins taken

FINAL CALORIES
(Calories eaten - calories burned)

Change? +/-

Date _______________________

How are you feeling today? _______________________

| **I have eaten...** | **I have exercised...** |

I have eaten...

BREAKFAST	**WHAT TIME?**	Calories

LUNCH	**WHAT TIME?**	Calories

DINNER	**WHAT TIME?**	Calories

SNACKS	**WHAT TIME?**	Calories

TOTAL CALORIES _______________________

Weight today? _______________________

I have exercised...

DOING?	**TIME**	Calories Burned

TOTAL CALORIES BURNED _______________________

I have slept...

_______________________ HOURS

I have drank...

CUPS OF WATER

Meds/vitamins taken

FINAL CALORIES _______________________
(Calories eaten - calories burned)

Change? +/- _______________________

Date _______________

How are you feeling today? _______________

I have eaten...

BREAKFAST	WHAT TIME?	Calories

LUNCH	WHAT TIME?	Calories

DINNER	WHAT TIME?	Calories

SNACKS	WHAT TIME?	Calories

TOTAL CALORIES _______________

Weight today? _______________

I have exercised...

DOING?	TIME	Calories Burned

TOTAL CALORIES BURNED _______________

I have slept...

_______________ HOURS

I have drank...

_______________ CUPS OF WATER

Meds/vitamins taken

FINAL CALORIES _______________

(Calories eaten - calories burned)

Change? +/- _______________

Date

How are you feeling today?

I have eaten...

BREAKFAST	**WHAT TIME?**	Calories

LUNCH	**WHAT TIME?**	Calories

DINNER	**WHAT TIME?**	Calories

SNACKS	**WHAT TIME?**	Calories

TOTAL CALORIES

Weight today?

I have exercised...

DOING?	**TIME**	Calories Burned

**TOTAL CALORIES
BURNED**

I have slept...

HOURS

I have drank...

CUPS OF
WATER

Meds/vitamins taken

FINAL CALORIES
(Calories eaten - calories burned)

Change? +/-

Date

How are you feeling today?

I have eaten...

BREAKFAST   **WHAT TIME?**   Calories

LUNCH   **WHAT TIME?**   Calories

DINNER   **WHAT TIME?**   Calories

SNACKS   **WHAT TIME?**   Calories

TOTAL CALORIES

Weight today?

I have exercised...

DOING?   **TIME**   Calories Burned

**TOTAL CALORIES
BURNED**

I have slept...

HOURS

I have drank...

CUPS OF
WATER

Meds/vitamins taken

FINAL CALORIES
(Calories eaten - calories burned)

Change? +/-

Date _______________

How are you feeling today? _______________

I have eaten...

BREAKFAST	**WHAT TIME?**	Calories

LUNCH	**WHAT TIME?**	Calories

DINNER	**WHAT TIME?**	Calories

SNACKS	**WHAT TIME?**	Calories

TOTAL CALORIES _______________

Weight today? _______________

I have exercised...

DOING?	**TIME**	Calories Burned

TOTAL CALORIES BURNED _______________

I have slept...

_______________ HOURS

I have drank...

_______________ CUPS OF WATER

Meds/vitamins taken

____

FINAL CALORIES _______________
(Calories eaten - calories burned)

Change? +/- _______________

Date

How are you feeling today?

I have eaten...

BREAKFAST	WHAT TIME?	Calories

LUNCH	WHAT TIME?	Calories

DINNER	WHAT TIME?	Calories

SNACKS	WHAT TIME?	Calories

TOTAL CALORIES

Weight today?

I have exercised...

DOING?	TIME	Calories Burned

TOTAL CALORIES BURNED

I have slept...

HOURS

I have drank...

CUPS OF WATER

Meds/vitamins taken

FINAL CALORIES

(Calories eaten - calories burned)

Change? +/-

Date

How are you feeling today?

I have eaten...

BREAKFAST	WHAT TIME?	Calories

LUNCH	WHAT TIME?	Calories

DINNER	WHAT TIME?	Calories

SNACKS	WHAT TIME?	Calories

TOTAL CALORIES

Weight today?

I have exercised...

DOING?	TIME	Calories Burned

TOTAL CALORIES BURNED

I have slept...

HOURS

I have drank...

CUPS OF WATER

Meds/vitamins taken

FINAL CALORIES
(Calories eaten - calories burned)

Change? +/-

Date

How are you feeling today?

I have eaten...

BREAKFAST	**WHAT TIME?**	Calories

LUNCH	**WHAT TIME?**	Calories

DINNER	**WHAT TIME?**	Calories

SNACKS	**WHAT TIME?**	Calories

TOTAL CALORIES

Weight today?

I have exercised...

DOING?	**TIME**	Calories Burned

TOTAL CALORIES BURNED

I have slept...

HOURS

I have drank...

CUPS OF WATER

Meds/vitamins taken

FINAL CALORIES
(Calories eaten - calories burned)

Change? +/-

Date

How are you feeling today?

I have eaten...

BREAKFAST	**WHAT TIME?**	Calories

LUNCH	**WHAT TIME?**	Calories

DINNER	**WHAT TIME?**	Calories

SNACKS	**WHAT TIME?**	Calories

TOTAL CALORIES

Weight today?

I have exercised...

DOING?	**TIME**	Calories Burned

TOTAL CALORIES BURNED

I have slept...

HOURS

I have drank...

CUPS OF WATER

Meds/vitamins taken

FINAL CALORIES
(Calories eaten - calories burned)

Change? +/-

Date _______________________

How are you feeling today? _______________________

# I have eaten...			# I have exercised...		
BREAKFAST	**WHAT TIME?**	Calories	DOING?	**TIME**	Calories Burned

TOTAL CALORIES BURNED _______________________

I have slept...

_______________________ HOURS

I have drank...

CUPS OF WATER _______________________

Meds/vitamins taken

TOTAL CALORIES _______________________

FINAL CALORIES _______________________
(Calories eaten - calories burned)

Weight today? _______________________

Change? +/- _______________________

Date _______________

How are you feeling today? _______________

I have eaten...

BREAKFAST	**WHAT TIME?**	Calories

LUNCH	**WHAT TIME?**	Calories

DINNER	**WHAT TIME?**	Calories

SNACKS	**WHAT TIME?**	Calories

TOTAL CALORIES _______________

Weight today? _______________

I have exercised...

DOING?	**TIME**	Calories Burned

TOTAL CALORIES BURNED _______________

I have slept...

_______________ HOURS

I have drank...

_______________ CUPS OF WATER

Meds/vitamins taken

____
____
____
____

FINAL CALORIES _______________
(Calories eaten - calories burned)

Change? +/- _______________

Date _______________________

How are you feeling today? _______________________

I have eaten...

BREAKFAST	**WHAT TIME?**	Calories

LUNCH	**WHAT TIME?**	Calories

DINNER	**WHAT TIME?**	Calories

SNACKS	**WHAT TIME?**	Calories

TOTAL CALORIES _______________________

Weight today? _______________________

I have exercised...

DOING?	**TIME**	Calories Burned

TOTAL CALORIES BURNED _______________________

I have slept...

_______________________ HOURS

I have drank...

_______________________ CUPS OF WATER

Meds/vitamins taken

FINAL CALORIES _______________________
(Calories eaten - calories burned)

Change? +/- _______________________

Date

How are you feeling today?

I have eaten...

BREAKFAST	WHAT TIME?	Calories

LUNCH	WHAT TIME?	Calories

DINNER	WHAT TIME?	Calories

SNACKS	WHAT TIME?	Calories

TOTAL CALORIES

Weight today?

I have exercised...

DOING?	TIME	Calories Burned

TOTAL CALORIES BURNED

I have slept...

HOURS

I have drank...

CUPS OF WATER

Meds/vitamins taken

FINAL CALORIES
(Calories eaten - calories burned)

Change? +/-

Date _______________

How are you feeling today? _______________

I have eaten...

BREAKFAST	**WHAT TIME?**	Calories

LUNCH	**WHAT TIME?**	Calories

DINNER	**WHAT TIME?**	Calories

SNACKS	**WHAT TIME?**	Calories

TOTAL CALORIES _______________

I have exercised...

DOING?	**TIME**	Calories Burned

TOTAL CALORIES BURNED _______________

I have slept...

_______________ HOURS

I have drank...

_______________ CUPS OF WATER

Meds/vitamins taken

____

FINAL CALORIES _______________
(Calories eaten - calories burned)

Weight today? _______________

Change? +/- _______________

Date

How are you feeling today?

I have eaten...

BREAKFAST	WHAT TIME?	Calories

LUNCH	WHAT TIME?	Calories

DINNER	WHAT TIME?	Calories

SNACKS	WHAT TIME?	Calories

TOTAL CALORIES

Weight today?

I have exercised...

DOING?	TIME	Calories Burned

TOTAL CALORIES BURNED

I have slept...

HOURS

I have drank...

CUPS OF WATER

Meds/vitamins taken

FINAL CALORIES
(Calories eaten - calories burned)

Change? +/-

Date _______________

How are you feeling today? _______________

I have eaten...

BREAKFAST	WHAT TIME?	Calories

LUNCH	WHAT TIME?	Calories

DINNER	WHAT TIME?	Calories

SNACKS	WHAT TIME?	Calories

TOTAL CALORIES _______________

Weight today? _______________

I have exercised...

DOING?	TIME	Calories Burned

TOTAL CALORIES BURNED _______________

I have slept...

_______________ HOURS

I have drank...

_______________ CUPS OF WATER

Meds/vitamins taken

____
____
____
____

FINAL CALORIES _______________
(Calories eaten - calories burned)

Change? +/- _______________

Date

How are you feeling today?

I have eaten...

| BREAKFAST | **WHAT TIME?** | Calories |

| LUNCH | **WHAT TIME?** | Calories |

| DINNER | **WHAT TIME?** | Calories |

| SNACKS | **WHAT TIME?** | Calories |

TOTAL CALORIES

Weight today?

I have exercised...

| DOING? | **TIME** | Calories Burned |

**TOTAL CALORIES
BURNED**

I have slept...

HOURS

I have drank...

CUPS OF
WATER

Meds/vitamins taken

FINAL CALORIES
(Calories eaten - calories burned)

Change? +/-

Date

How are you feeling today?

I have eaten...

BREAKFAST	**WHAT TIME?**	Calories

LUNCH	**WHAT TIME?**	Calories

DINNER	**WHAT TIME?**	Calories

SNACKS	**WHAT TIME?**	Calories

TOTAL CALORIES

Weight today?

I have exercised...

DOING?	**TIME**	Calories Burned

TOTAL CALORIES BURNED

I have slept...

HOURS

I have drank...

CUPS OF WATER

Meds/vitamins taken

FINAL CALORIES

(Calories eaten - calories burned)

Change? +/-

SIMPLE WEIGHT TRACKER

DATE	TIME	WEIGHT	NOTES / COMMENTS

SIMPLE WEIGHT TRACKER

DATE	TIME	WEIGHT	NOTES / COMMENTS

SIMPLE WEIGHT TRACKER

DATE	TIME	WEIGHT	NOTES / COMMENTS

SIMPLE WEIGHT TRACKER

DATE	TIME	WEIGHT	NOTES / COMMENTS

SIMPLE WEIGHT TRACKER

DATE	TIME	WEIGHT	NOTES / COMMENTS

SIMPLE WEIGHT TRACKER

DATE	TIME	WEIGHT	NOTES / COMMENTS

SIMPLE WEIGHT TRACKER

DATE	TIME	WEIGHT	NOTES / COMMENTS

SIMPLE WEIGHT TRACKER

DATE	TIME	WEIGHT	NOTES / COMMENTS

SIMPLE WEIGHT TRACKER

DATE	TIME	WEIGHT	NOTES / COMMENTS

SIMPLE WEIGHT TRACKER

DATE	TIME	WEIGHT	NOTES / COMMENTS

Monday	Breakfast	Lunch	Dinner

Tuesday	Breakfast	Lunch	Dinner

Wednesday	Breakfast	Lunch	Dinner

Thursday	Breakfast	Lunch	Dinner

Friday	Breakfast	Lunch	Dinner

Saturday	Breakfast	Lunch	Dinner

Sunday	Breakfast	Lunch	Dinner

	Breakfast	Lunch	Dinner
Monday			

	Breakfast	Lunch	Dinner
Tuesday			

	Breakfast	Lunch	Dinner
Wednesday			

	Breakfast	Lunch	Dinner
Thursday			

	Breakfast	Lunch	Dinner
Friday			

	Breakfast	Lunch	Dinner
Saturday			

	Breakfast	Lunch	Dinner
Sunday			

Monday	Breakfast	Lunch	Dinner

Tuesday	Breakfast	Lunch	Dinner

Wednesday	Breakfast	Lunch	Dinner

Thursday	Breakfast	Lunch	Dinner

Friday	Breakfast	Lunch	Dinner

Saturday	Breakfast	Lunch	Dinner

Sunday	Breakfast	Lunch	Dinner

	Breakfast	Lunch	Dinner
Monday			

	Breakfast	Lunch	Dinner
Tuesday			

	Breakfast	Lunch	Dinner
Wednesday			

	Breakfast	Lunch	Dinner
Thursday			

	Breakfast	Lunch	Dinner
Friday			

	Breakfast	Lunch	Dinner
Saturday			

	Breakfast	Lunch	Dinner
Sunday			

Monday	Breakfast	Lunch	Dinner

Tuesday	Breakfast	Lunch	Dinner

Wednesday	Breakfast	Lunch	Dinner

Thursday	Breakfast	Lunch	Dinner

Friday	Breakfast	Lunch	Dinner

Saturday	Breakfast	Lunch	Dinner

Sunday	Breakfast	Lunch	Dinner

Monday	Breakfast	Lunch	Dinner

Tuesday	Breakfast	Lunch	Dinner

Wednesday	Breakfast	Lunch	Dinner

Thursday	Breakfast	Lunch	Dinner

Friday	Breakfast	Lunch	Dinner

Saturday	Breakfast	Lunch	Dinner

Sunday	Breakfast	Lunch	Dinner

Monday	Breakfast	Lunch	Dinner

Tuesday	Breakfast	Lunch	Dinner

Wednesday	Breakfast	Lunch	Dinner

Thursday	Breakfast	Lunch	Dinner

Friday	Breakfast	Lunch	Dinner

Saturday	Breakfast	Lunch	Dinner

Sunday	Breakfast	Lunch	Dinner

Monday	Breakfast	Lunch	Dinner

Tuesday	Breakfast	Lunch	Dinner

Wednesday	Breakfast	Lunch	Dinner

Thursday	Breakfast	Lunch	Dinner

Friday	Breakfast	Lunch	Dinner

Saturday	Breakfast	Lunch	Dinner

Sunday	Breakfast	Lunch	Dinner

Monday	Breakfast	Lunch	Dinner

Tuesday	Breakfast	Lunch	Dinner

Wednesday	Breakfast	Lunch	Dinner

Thursday	Breakfast	Lunch	Dinner

Friday	Breakfast	Lunch	Dinner

Saturday	Breakfast	Lunch	Dinner

Sunday	Breakfast	Lunch	Dinner

Monday	Breakfast	Lunch	Dinner

Tuesday	Breakfast	Lunch	Dinner

Wednesday	Breakfast	Lunch	Dinner

Thursday	Breakfast	Lunch	Dinner

Friday	Breakfast	Lunch	Dinner

Saturday	Breakfast	Lunch	Dinner

Sunday	Breakfast	Lunch	Dinner

Monday	Breakfast	Lunch	Dinner

Tuesday	Breakfast	Lunch	Dinner

Wednesday	Breakfast	Lunch	Dinner

Thursday	Breakfast	Lunch	Dinner

Friday	Breakfast	Lunch	Dinner

Saturday	Breakfast	Lunch	Dinner

Sunday	Breakfast	Lunch	Dinner

Monday	Breakfast	Lunch	Dinner

Tuesday	Breakfast	Lunch	Dinner

Wednesday	Breakfast	Lunch	Dinner

Thursday	Breakfast	Lunch	Dinner

Friday	Breakfast	Lunch	Dinner

Saturday	Breakfast	Lunch	Dinner

Sunday	Breakfast	Lunch	Dinner

Monday	Breakfast	Lunch	Dinner

Tuesday	Breakfast	Lunch	Dinner

Wednesday	Breakfast	Lunch	Dinner

Thursday	Breakfast	Lunch	Dinner

Friday	Breakfast	Lunch	Dinner

Saturday	Breakfast	Lunch	Dinner

Sunday	Breakfast	Lunch	Dinner

	Breakfast	Lunch	Dinner
Monday			
Tuesday			
Wednesday			
Thursday			
Friday			
Saturday			
Sunday			

Monday	Breakfast	Lunch	Dinner

Tuesday	Breakfast	Lunch	Dinner

Wednesday	Breakfast	Lunch	Dinner

Thursday	Breakfast	Lunch	Dinner

Friday	Breakfast	Lunch	Dinner

Saturday	Breakfast	Lunch	Dinner

Sunday	Breakfast	Lunch	Dinner

Monday	Breakfast	Lunch	Dinner

Tuesday	Breakfast	Lunch	Dinner

Wednesday	Breakfast	Lunch	Dinner

Thursday	Breakfast	Lunch	Dinner

Friday	Breakfast	Lunch	Dinner

Saturday	Breakfast	Lunch	Dinner

Sunday	Breakfast	Lunch	Dinner

Monday	Breakfast	Lunch	Dinner

Tuesday	Breakfast	Lunch	Dinner

Wednesday	Breakfast	Lunch	Dinner

Thursday	Breakfast	Lunch	Dinner

Friday	Breakfast	Lunch	Dinner

Saturday	Breakfast	Lunch	Dinner

Sunday	Breakfast	Lunch	Dinner

Monday	Breakfast	Lunch	Dinner

Tuesday	Breakfast	Lunch	Dinner

Wednesday	Breakfast	Lunch	Dinner

Thursday	Breakfast	Lunch	Dinner

Friday	Breakfast	Lunch	Dinner

Saturday	Breakfast	Lunch	Dinner

Sunday	Breakfast	Lunch	Dinner

Monday	Breakfast	Lunch	Dinner

Tuesday	Breakfast	Lunch	Dinner

Wednesday	Breakfast	Lunch	Dinner

Thursday	Breakfast	Lunch	Dinner

Friday	Breakfast	Lunch	Dinner

Saturday	Breakfast	Lunch	Dinner

Sunday	Breakfast	Lunch	Dinner

Monday	Breakfast	Lunch	Dinner

Tuesday	Breakfast	Lunch	Dinner

Wednesday	Breakfast	Lunch	Dinner

Thursday	Breakfast	Lunch	Dinner

Friday	Breakfast	Lunch	Dinner

Saturday	Breakfast	Lunch	Dinner

Sunday	Breakfast	Lunch	Dinner

	Breakfast	Lunch	Dinner
Monday			

	Breakfast	Lunch	Dinner
Tuesday			

	Breakfast	Lunch	Dinner
Wednesday			

	Breakfast	Lunch	Dinner
Thursday			

	Breakfast	Lunch	Dinner
Friday			

	Breakfast	Lunch	Dinner
Saturday			

	Breakfast	Lunch	Dinner
Sunday			

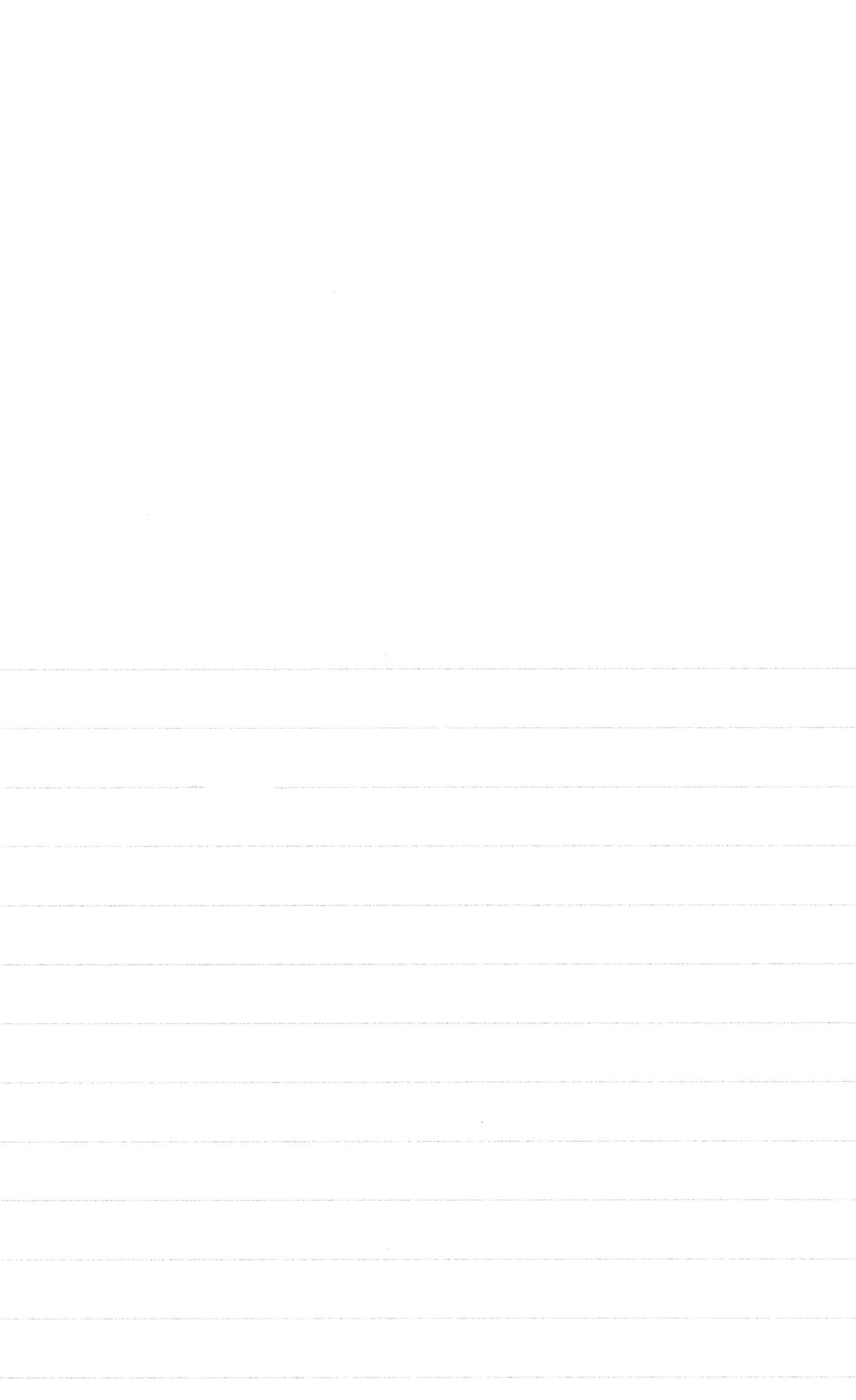

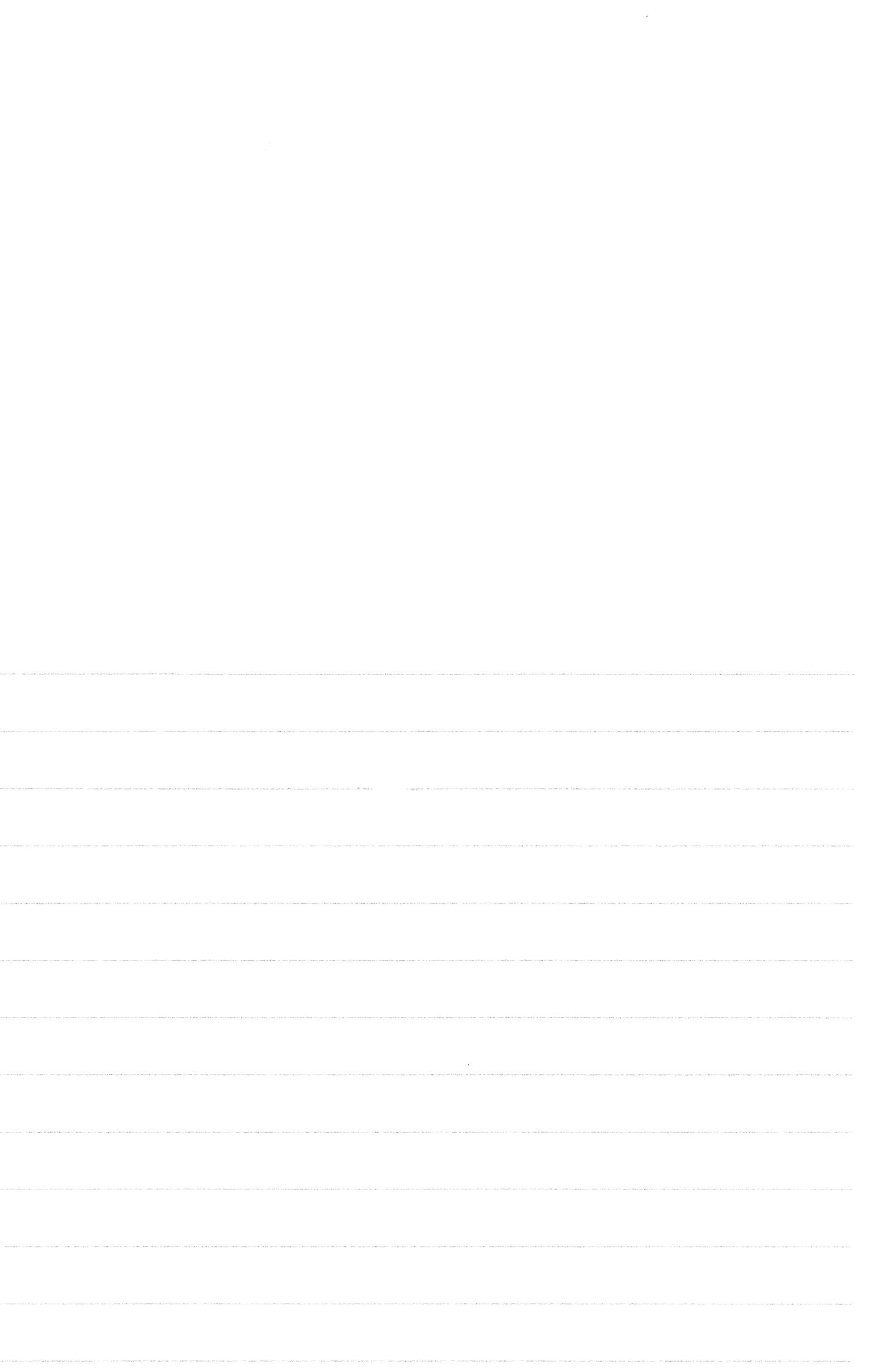

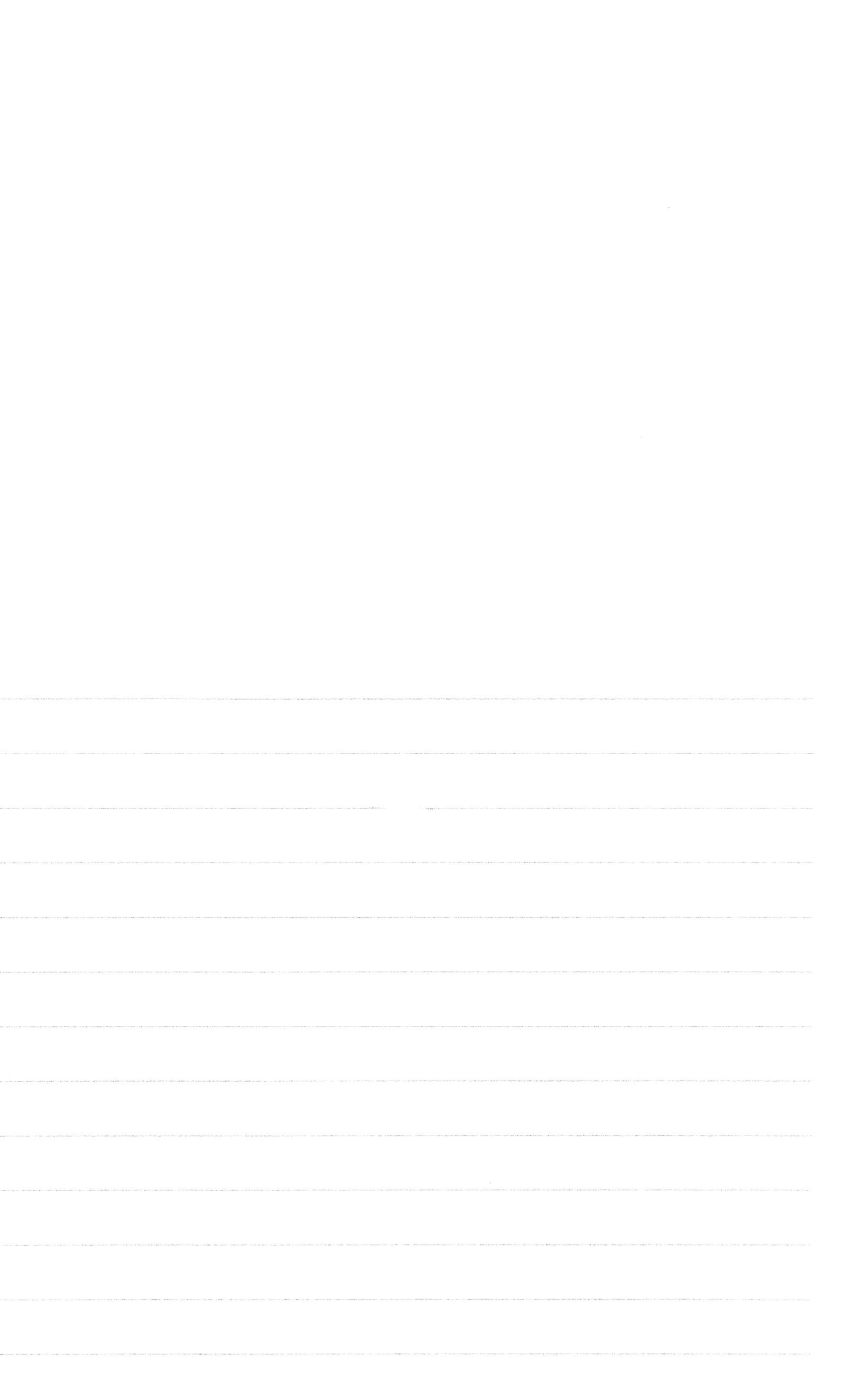